PET IN

PET PHOTO

NAME	
DOB	
BREED	
GENDER	
COLOR	
MICROCHIP	
BREED REGISTRATION	
BLOOD TYPE	

PET OWNER

PET OWNER PHOTO

NAME	
SURNAME	
ADDRESS	
POSTCODE	
CITY	
COUNTRY	
TELEPHONE NUMBER	
MAIL	

IMPORTANT CONTACTS

Veterinarian	
Vet Address	
Vet Contact	
Vet Mail	
Emergency VET	
Groomer	
Pet Sitter	
Others	

PHYSICAL OBSERVATIONS

Date	Weight	Height/Length	Physical Observations

PHYSICAL OBSERVATIONS

Date	Weight	Height/Length	Physical Observations

VACCINATION RECORDS

VACCINE	IMMUNIZATION DATE				VETERINARIAN

VACCINATION RECORDS

VACCINE	IMMUNIZATION DATE				VETERINARIAN

MEDICAL TREATMENTS

Date	Treatment	Notes

MEDICAL TREATMENTS

Date	Treatment	Notes

Made in United States
Troutdale, OR
12/20/2024

26912527R00056